The Compl Diet Cookbook

A Quick Guide to Delicious Paleo Recipes

Charlie Mason

CONTENTS

INTRODUCTION

Congratulations and thank you so much for purchasing The Complete Paleo Diet Cookbook!

This book is loaded with a variety of delicious recipes that will keep you on the right track as you begin your journey amongst your cavemen ancestors via the Paleo Diet. This is the perfect starter cookbook for those beginning the Paleo Diet. All the recipes are simple and easy-to-make in the comfort of your own kitchen.

So what are you waiting for? It's time to dive into the chapters full of recipes and get to cooking!

CHAPTER 1: BREAKFAST

Breakfast Egg Muffins

This is a delightful, low carb, free-range recipe that will give you a great boost for the morning, without weighing you down. This recipe is just eggs and veggies, so no carb-loaded bread to make you feel sluggish. This is great to store and have to grab for a quick breakfast on the go. This recipe makes about twelve muffins. One muffin equals one serving, so roughly twelve servings, depending on how many veggies you add to the eggs.

Ingredients:
• 12 free-range, organic eggs. (Home raised chickens produce the best eggs for this)
• Tsp of coconut oil. (Could also use grass-fed butter or organic olive oil)
• Veggies. (How many depends on the kind you use.)

Instructions
• Preheat your oven to 350 degrees Fahrenheit. While the oven is preheating, lightly grease your muffin tin. This prevents the eggs from sticking, to allow for easy removal.
• Whisk your eggs in a bowl, and add veggies. Ration your eggs into separate bowls if making different veggie combinations. Pour eggs evenly into muffin tins.
• Bake for 20-25 minutes or until eggs have set.
• That was easy! If you are looking for a little more seasoning, you can add whatever seasonings you like, just make sure to watch sodium levels. You can also top with things like avocado, and peppers. This is a lovely, versatile, and simple recipe.

Apple Cider Donuts
This is a lovely breakfast idea for those days where you are craving the

wonderful taste of donuts, but you don't want to break your diet. This adheres to the rules of the diet, but is still packed with wonderful flavor and will satisfy your cravings.

Ingredients
- 1/2 c. coconut flour
- 1/2 tsp cinnamon
- 1/2 tsp baking soda
- 1/8 tsp celtic sea salt
- 2 organic eggs (unchilled)
- 2 tbsp honey
- 2 tbsp coconut oil (melted)
- 1/2 c. warm apple cider
- 2 tbsp ghee (This will be used to adhere the sugar when you are coating the donuts)

For the Cinnamon Sugar
- 1/2 c. granulated coconut sugar
- 1 tbsp cinnamon

Instructions
- Preheat a mini donut maker
- In a bowl, about medium sized, whisk together eggs, oil, and honey.
- Add the dry ingredients to the wet ingredients and stir until combined.
- Then you add the warm apple cider to the mixture until its well incorporated into the dough.
- Get a cookie scooper, and scoop the batter into the donut maker that you have preheated.
- The donuts should be cooked in two to three minutes.
- Remove the pastries from the maker and place on a cooling rack to brush them with your glaze of choice.
- Toss donuts with the prepared cinnamon/coconut sugar mixture until they are well coated.
- This is not only a great breakfast piece, but it is also good for a romantic gesture to your partner. Breakfast in bed without the mess. Who doesn't love that?

Apple Muffins

The Paleo diet is often lacking in true muffins. However, for people who are busy and on the go, muffins provide a great energy boost to get you through the day.

Ingredients
- 2 c. almond flour (also known as almond meal)
- 3 organic eggs
- 2 tbsp melted, grass-fed butter
- 2 tbsp - 1/4 c honey (to taste)
- 2 tsp ground cinnamon
- 1 or 2 apples. Core and chop them into a blender
- 1 tsp baking soda
- just a pinch of sea salt

Instructions
- Preheat your oven to 325 degrees Fahrenheit, and start your prep work. First core, and chop your apples until finely blended, but not pureed. This will get them to the perfect texture for the muffins.
- To prepare muffins, simply whisk together all of the ingredients into a bowl. Then fill a greased muffin tin evenly. Each cup should be about 3/4 full to allow room for batter expansion.
- It is easy to whip these together on a Sunday, and have them stored in a fridge for a busy week. This way you do not have to skip out on breakfast. A lot of people use the excuse that they are too busy to eat breakfast, but if you prep properly you should never have to skip the most important meal of the day.
- Be careful though, if you cook these all the way through, they could be a little dry. This is great if you like a drier muffin, however, if you like moist, pull them from the oven when the toothpick comes out only mostly clean. They will finish cooking up as they cool, and not be as dry.
- What is breakfast without a smoothie? Here are two smoothies that will rock your morning routine. All are power packed to give you a boost and keep you from the midday jitters.

Avocado, Kale, and Peach Smoothie

Ingredients
- 1/2 to 1 ripened avocado
- 1/2 a banana (you can use frozen or fresh)
- 3 or 4 peach slices (you can use fresh or frozen)
- 1/4 to 1/2 c. kale, frozen and chopped finely
- 1 c almond milk. Can also use it coconut milk and almond milk blend.

Instructions
- Throw all of the ingredients in your blender, and blend until they have reached the consistency you desire.
- If you are using frozen fruits, it is essential to make sure you use the ones without added sugar. This is a milder smoothie, so if you want to sweeten it up, use some raw honey or agave. It tastes almost like a cucumber without it, despite the fact that there are no cucumbers in the smoothie.
- Most people scoff at the thought of avocado in the smoothie, but the truth is that it is great smoothie material. It gives the smoothie a light and airy texture, and its healthy fats keep you full till lunch, so you won't be crashing before then.

Strawberry, Spinach, and Almond Butter Smoothie

Ingredients
- 1 c. almond milk (you can mix almond and coconut milk for a richer flavor)
- 1/4-1/2 c. Chopped and frozen spinach
- 3-4 lg. strawberries (Fresh or from the freezer isle)
- 1/2 banana (fresh or from the freezer isle)
- 2-3 tbsp almond butter

Instructions

• Pour all ingredients into a blender and blend till you achieve desired texture.

• Frozen fruits tend to be easier to keep on hand, as the worry of spoiling is reduced. However, you have to read the labels and make sure that there are no added sugars. Also, a mixture of coconut and almond milk give the smoothie a richer texture, as coconut milk tends to be a little thin.

• Almond butter is a great source of protein and healthy fats, in order to give you a boost throughout the day.

No Fail Paleo Pancakes

This is an easy-peazy recipe that is perfect for Paleo folks who do not have ample time in the A.M. to whip up breakfast!

Ingredients

• 1 tsp. vanilla extract
• 1 tsp. cinnamon
• 1 tbsp. coconut flour
• 2 eggs
• 1 banana
• Dark chocolate chips, fruit you desire, and/or maple syrup, for serving.

Instructions

• Mash your banana, then mix with vanilla, cinnamon, coconut flour, and eggs.

• Warm up pan. Pour batter into pan, creating 3 evenly sized pancakes.

• Add in optional toppings.

• Cook 2-4 minutes on first side, flip, and cook 2 minutes on opposing side.

• Drizzle with syrup and enjoy!

Sweet Potato and Bacon Breakfast Fritters

Ingredients
- Pepper and salt
- 1 tsp. paprika
- 3 tbsp. coconut flour
- 2 whisked eggs
- 3 chopped scallions
- 2 peeled sweet potatoes
- 6 strips of bacon

Instructions
- Slice bacon into ½" pieces. Fry in pan till crispy. Remove and reserve bacon fat.
- Peel and grate potatoes. Pour shredded sweet potatoes into a bowl. Mix with pepper, salt, coconut flour, eggs, scallions, and cooked bacon pieces.
- Using a ¼ measuring cup, scoop out fritter mixture. Plop mixture onto parchment paper, and flatten with spatula to form fritter. You want them to be about ¾" thick.
- Add olive oil to pan along with bacon fat and heat up.
- Cook 3-4 fritters for 3 minutes per side till golden. Serve warm!

Paleo Crepes with Strawberries

Ingredients
Strawberry Sauce:
- 2 tsp. arrowroot
- ½ C. water
- 1 tbsp. honey
- 2 tbsp. coconut sugar
- 8 ounces strawberries

Crepes:
- ½ C. canned coconut milk
- 1 tsp. Honey
- 1 tsp. vanilla extract
- 3 eggs
- 1/3 C. arrowroot
- 1/3 C. coconut flour

Coconut Whipped Cream:
- 1 can full-fat coconut milk, chilled

Instructions
- To make sauce, add chopped strawberries and honey to pan. Mix in arrowroot powder with cold water. Heat till boiling, then turn down heat and simmer 5-10 minutes till thickened.
- To make crepes, mix coconut milk, eggs, honey, vanilla, and flours together. Let sit 5 minutes. Heat skillet with a bit of olive oil. Pour crepe batter into center of pan, swirl and let cook 1-2 minutes. Flip and cook 30 seconds more.
- To make coconut whipped cream, pour coconut cream into mixer along with 1-3 drops of vanilla extract. Whisk till thick. Add more vanilla or honey if you wish.
- Line strawberries on crepe along with a spoon of whipped cream. Roll crepe. Serve right away with leftover whipped cream. Enjoy!

CHAPTER 2: LUNCH

Lunch, while almost always eaten, is kind of treated as a joke. There are rarely any specified lunch recipes that don't involve a sandwich of some sort. Most people either make a sandwich or eat leftovers, and with carbs being a no-no in the paleo diet, then the sandwiches are out. This can make it seem like the options are limited. However, this chapter has a bunch of great ideas that can be prepped the night before.

Chipotle Chicken Lettuce Wraps

Don't laugh. If you had only had wimpy lettuce wraps that left you hungrier than you were before you ate, then you are in for a treat. This lettuce wrap is packed with flavors enough to satisfy your taste-buds, and fulfilling enough to get you through your day.

Ingredients
• 1c of chicken breast (skinless). Chunked, shredded, or cut into strips
• 2 tbsp olive oil
• 1 finely sliced red onion
• 1 large ripe tomato, chopped.
• 1 tbsp of chipotle in adobo sauce
• 1/2 tsp cumin
• Pinch of salt, pepper, and brown sugar.
• Choice of lettuce leaves
• coriander leaves, fresh
• jalapenos, pickled and fresh
• Avacodo or fresh guacamole
• Tomatoes, scallions, onion, and other ingredients that could be used to make a rustic salsa
• lime wedges to spritz

Instructions
• Heat your oil in a nonstick pan over a medium heat and cook your chicken until it is golden brown.

- Then, add another splash of oil, and sauté your onions
- Add the rest of the ingredients minus the lime, salad ingredients, and lettuce, and simmer for about ten to fifteen minutes.
- Add the chicken back in and simmer for about five more minutes.
- Store the mixture in a bowl, and place the lettuce and other elements in another bowl, and make for lunch the next day.
- Before eating, if you wish, spritz the wrap with lime.
- Lettuce wraps have all of the flavors of a regular wrap, without the carbs of the tortilla.

California Turkey and Bacon Wrap with Basil Mayo

If you like California inspired food, you would love this recipe. Satisfy your taste buds with the delicious combination of basil flavored mayo, bacon and turkey. This is every paleo lover's dream lunch. Who says lettuce wraps have to be boring and bland?

Ingredients
- 6 fresh basil leaves
- 1/2 c. mayo
- 1 tsp lemon juice,
- 1 clove garlic
- salt and pepper
- 4 bacon slices
- iceberg lettuce
- turkey slices

Instructions
- Start with the basil- mayo. Throw the first six ingredients in a food processor and blend until they reach a creamy consistency.
- You want your bacon to be slightly floppy, so it manipulates well in the wrap. This means you need to microwave the bacon on a bed of paper towels. You can go anywhere between five and seven

minutes. This should give you a good texture to your bacon.

• You can use whatever kind of lettuce you would like, however Iceberg lettuce seems to give the biggest leaves, and that keeps everything less messy. Messy wraps can be frustrating, so you want to avoid them at all costs.

• You want the wrap to stay crunchy, and the basil mayo can make the lettuce soggy, so you want a barrier. Take one turkey slice, and lay it on the lettuce, then add the mayo. Finally, top with one more turkey slice, and add the bacon. Roll up, and enjoy!

BBQ Chicken and Roasted Sweet Potato Bowls

Ingredients
• ½ C. BBQ sauce
• 1 pound boneless skinless chicken breasts
• 1 head of broccoli
• ½ tsp. chili powder
• ½ tsp. garlic powder
• ½ tsp. salt
• 2 tbsp. olive oil
• 1 yellow onion
• 2 sweet potatoes

Instructions
• Ensure oven is preheated to 400 degrees Fahrenheit. With foil, line a pan.

• Peel and slice sweet potatoes. Then slice potatoes and onion into chunks. Pour onto pan and toss with 1 tablespoon olive oil. Then sprinkle with chili powder, garlic powder, and ¼ teaspoon salt.

• Toss well and add broccoli. Then sprinkle remaining olive oil and salt.

• Place breasts onto pan among veggies and brush with ¼ cup of BBQ sauce.

• Bake 15-20 minutes till chicken is cooked completely.

- Take pan from oven and shred chicken. Toss shredded meat with remaining BBQ sauce.
- Place chicken and roasted veggies in bowls. Enjoy this healthy lunch!

Strawberry Mango Salad

Ingredients
Strawberry Poppy Seed Dressing:
- ¼ tsp. salt
- 1 tbsp. poppy seeds
- ½ C. strawberries
- ¼ C. honey
- 1/3 C. champagne vinegar
- ½ C. olive oil

Strawberry Mango Salad:
- 1 C. sliced/roasted almonds
- 1 chopped avocado
- 1 C. chopped strawberries
- 1 chopped mango
- 2 8-ounce cooked/chopped chicken breasts
- 8 C. baby greens

Instructions
- To make dressing, pour all dressing ingredients into a blender and blend till everything is smooth.
- To create salad, combine all salad ingredients in a large bowl, tossing gently. Toss with dressing and serve!

Creamy Cauliflower Soup

Ingredients
- ½ tsp. smoked paprika
- 1 tsp. onion powder
- ¾ tsp. dried chives
- 2 tsp. salt
- 1 sprig rosemary
- 32 ounces chicken broth
- 1 head cauliflower
- 4 slices cloves of garlic
- ½ sliced yellow onion
- 2 tbsp. ghee
- 2 ounces cubed pancetta, to serve

Instructions
- Add ghee, garlic cloves, and onion to a pre-heated pan. Sauté together 60 seconds till mixture becomes fragrant.
- Place rosemary, broth, cauliflower florets and half of salt into pan. Cover and turn down heat to simmer 25 minutes till cauliflower becomes tender.
- As cauliflower mixture cooks, saute pancetta till crisp. Put on paper towel lined plate.
- Once cauliflower is tender, take out rosemary and pour in remaining salt, herbs, and spices. Combine thoroughly.
- Pour soup mixture into a blender. Blender 30 seconds till smooth.
- Pour into serving bowls and serve topped with crispy pancetta and chives.

Buffalo Chicken Slides
Ingredients

- ¼ C. ranch dressing
- 1 large sweet potato
- ¼ tsp. pepper
- 2 tbsp. almond flour
- 2-3 tbsp. hot buffalo sauce
- 2 green onions
- 1 minced clove garlic
- 1 pound ground chicken

Instructions

- Ensure oven is preheated to 375 degrees Fahrenheit. With parchment paper, line a sheet.
- Slice sweet potato into ¼" rounds. Thinly slice both white and green parts of green onions.
- Place potato rounds in an even layer on sheet. Bake 15-20 minutes till lightly golden. Make sure to flip them halfway through bake time.
- Combine pepper, almond flour, buffalo sauce, green onions, garlic, and chicken together. Make 8 even portions from mixture with hands.
- Preheat grill. Flatten meat portions into patties. Grill 5 minutes per side.
- Arrange meat on potato rounds, using them as "buns." Serve with ranch.

Chicken and Zucchini Poppers
Ingredients

- ½ tsp. pepper
- 1 tsp. salt
- 1 clove of garlic

- 3-4 tbsp. minced cilantro
- 2-3 sliced green onions
- 2 C. grated zucchini
- 1 pound ground chicken breast
- ¾ tsp. cumin
- Olive oil

Instructions

- Toss pepper, salt, garlic, cilantro, green onion, zucchini, and chicken together.
- Heat up olive oil and add heaped tablespoons of zucchini mixture to pan. Cook 8-10 minutes, flip and cook 4-5 more minutes till golden brown and cooked through.

Fiesta Chicken Salad
Ingredients

- Pepper and salt
- Pinch of cayenne pepper
- ¼ tsp. smoked paprika
- ¼ tsp. cumin
- Juice of 1 lime
- 2 sliced scallions
- ¼ C. cilantro
- ½ red pepper, diced
- 2 C. cooked chicken (shredded or chopped)
- 1 avocado

Instructions

- Mash avocado.
- Mix remaining recipe components with avocado till thoroughly combined.
- Serve with favorite paleo sides!

CHAPTER 3: DINNER

Maple Pumpkin Meatballs

You are not blind. It really says Maple Pumpkin Meatballs. This is a great fall recipe for when you want to switch things up. This is a great recipe for Thanksgiving meatballs, to get all of your guests talking about the wonderful dish. You will have people asking your recipe, and they will never believe it is part of what most people call a "fad diet."

The maple and pumpkin give the meat a nice crisp taste, with just a hint of sweetness. This really makes them stand out, and they are moist and delightful as well.

Eat them by themselves, with some vegetti, on cauliflower rice, or however you please. They are delicious.

Ingredients
- 1 lb. Ground beef
- 1/2 lb. Ground pork
- 1/2 c. Pumpkin puree
- 1 organic Egg
- 1/2 c. Almond flour
- 1 minced, small onion
- 2 minced garlic cloves
- 1 minced, small bunch of parsley
- 1 tsp sea salt
- 1/2 tsp black pepper
- 1/4 c. Maple syrup

Instructions
- Heat your oven to 400 degrees Fahrenheit.
- Put all ingredients minus the syrup in a bowl, and get in there with your hands to combine them thoroughly.
- Throw some parchment paper down on a baking sheet, and roll your desired sized meatballs up and place on the baking sheet.
- Bake until thoroughly cooked and brown, about twenty to twenty-five minutes. Roll in maple syrup, and enjoy.

Chicken and Vegetable Bowl

Had a long day, and don't feel like cooking a major dinner, but don't want to break your diet? This is the recipe for you.

This recipe is simple, and it is healthy, you are pretty much consuming a rainbow.

Why is that important?

Every different color of fruits and veggies have a different nutrient in them. This means that when you eat a rainbow of variety, you are getting a ton of healthy nutrients. This will give you a good immune boost, and help you get through not only the night but the week as well.

These colors are called phytochemicals, and they take on the sun and break its properties down into different nutrients, which are called phytonutrients.

Phytonutrients help make up the certain vitamins that can be found in fruits and vegetables. In a very general sense, yellow and orange produce (like bell peppers and lemons) contain high amounts of vitamin A and vitamin C. Green veggies, and fruits contain vitamins B, E, and K while purple can signal the presence of vitamin C and K.

This salad will load down your bowl with all kinds of vitamins and minerals…and it tastes great too! What could be better?

Ingredients
- 3 tablespoons olive oil
- 2 cloves garlic minced
- 2 Bell peppers any color, sliced
- 1 Red onion sliced
- 4 cups Spinach chopped
- 1/2 cup shredded carrots
- 2 tablespoons Lemon juice
- 1/2 cup Chopped fresh parsley
- 2 cups cooked and shredded chicken breast
- Sprouts or microgreens for garnish
- Sea salt and fresh ground pepper to taste

Instructions
- Heat oil and throw all of the veggies but the sprouts in, and cook until softened.
- Add the chicken to the vegetables, and then cover with sprouts.

Spring Lamb Stir Fry

If you are sick of ground beef, then this is a good recipe to mix it up. Lamb is a whole new world and can make dinner exciting again.

This is such a good combination that you can eat it over cauliflower rice, or you can eat it alone just the lamb and veggies. Pair it with a tea to drink, or lemon ginger ale.

If you haven't had any experience with lamb, you should talk to your local grocer or butcher to find a lamb that is 100% organically fed, and grass fed. These two things are important to the diet.

Labeling laws mean that labels pretty much mean nothing. This means that as long as the animal is fed grass part of the time, they can label it grass-fed. This is something that can make it really confusing because you want 100% naturally raised livestock.

The reason it is so important is because non organically fed livestock are generally not as nutrient dense because they are fed hormones to make them larger, which means that the nutrients have to cover more area, and unless you buy the whole animal, you won't get the dense amount of nutrients. Organically fed animals are more nutrient dense, as they are typically slightly smaller, and they aren't getting their nutrients reduced from antibiotics and processed foods that just make the meat thicker.

A tender lamb is great for a springtime meal that isn't too filling, yet it is very satisfying. That may seem like a paradox, but the truth is, it fills your stomach without feeling heavy, like a lot of dinner meals would.

Ingredients
- 3 tbsp Coconut oil
- 1 lb. boneless lamb cubed
- 2 minced garlic cloves
- 1 tsp fresh ginger
- 2 sliced zucchini
- 1 sliced, large carrot
- 1 tsp Ground coriander
- 1 tsp Ground cumin
- 1 lime, juiced
- Cilantro, freshly chopped (to taste)
- 1 c. Cauliflower rice per serving
- salt and pepper to taste

Instructions
- Heat oil in a skillet on medium heat, and cook lamb until brown. Then, remove the lamb from the skillet, and toss in the veggies. Cook the veggies until they are just about soft, then add your lamb back to the pan.
- Cook the lamb until it is done, generally a medium rare is how lamb is served. Lay lamb and veggies on a bed of cauliflower rice, and top with cilantro. Season to taste.

Sweet and Spicy Chicken

Ingredients
- ½ C. oil
- 1 pound chicken

Sauce:
- Pinch of salt
- ½ tsp. apple cider vinegar
- ½ tsp ground ginger
- 1 tsp. garlic powder
- 5 tbsp. coconut amino
- ½ C. raw honey

Breading:
- 2 eggs + 1 tsp. water
- ¾ C. arrowroot flour

Other:
- Red pepper flakes
- Green onions
- 1 red bell pepper

Instructions

- Chop chicken into cubes.
- Mix all sauce ingredients together till incorporated. Then beat egg and water together. In another bowl, pour in arrowroot flour.
- Dip cubes of chicken into egg mixture first, then arrowroot flour.
- Heat oil in a pan.
- Put chicken cubes into pan, browning on all sides. Drain.
- Pour sauce over chicken and heat to boiling. Then turn down heat and simmer 10 minutes.
- Add slices of red bell pepper, diced green onions, and red pepper flakes, combing well. Serve!

Italian Spaghetti Squash Bake

Ingredients
Squash:

- ½ tsp. pepper
- ½ tsp. salt
- 2 tsp. extra-virgin olive oil
- 1 spaghetti squash

Other components:

- ½ tsp. salt
- ½ tsp. pepper
- 1 tbsp. garlic powder
- ½ tsp. red pepper flakes
- 1 ½ tbsp. Italian seasoning
- 1 egg
- 1 C. tomato sauce
- 1 pound boneless skinless chicken breasts (cooked and shredded)
- 3 handfuls spinach
- 1 crushed clove garlic

- 1 tsp. extra-virgin olive oil
- ¼ C. parmesan cheese, for serving

Instructions

- Ensure oven is preheated to 375 degrees Fahrenheit. With parchment, line a sheet.
- Slice squash in half and remove seeds. Drizzle with olive oil and sprinkle with pepper and salt. Place squash halves face side down onto sheet. Add ¼ cup water to sheet. Bake half an hour till tender.
- Scrape squash out with fork and place in bowl.
- Heat oil, and saute garlic. Then add spinach, cooking till it wilts.
- Mix shredded squash, cheese, egg, tomato sauce, shredded chicken, spinach, and garlic together. Pour into a dish. Sprinkle with parmesan and red pepper flakes.
- Bake 10 minutes. Then broil 3-5 minutes.

Harvest Chicken Skillet

Ingredients

- 1 C. chicken broth
- 1 tsp. cinnamon
- 2 tsp. thyme
- 4 minced cloves garlic
- 2 peeled/cored/cut Granny Smith apples
- 1 chopped onion
- 1 peeled/cut sweet potato
- 3 C. Brussels sprouts
- 4 chopped slices bacon
- ½ tsp. pepper
- 1 tsp. salt
- 1 pound boneless skinless chicken breasts, cubed
- 1 tbsp. olive oil

Instructions

- Heat oil and place chicken, ½ tsp salt and pepper. Cook till just browned. Put on plate and put to the side.
- Reduce heat and add bacon, cooking till crispy. Transfer to plate. Reserve 1 ½ tbsp. bacon fat.
- Increase heat and add remaining salt, onion, sweet potato, and Brussels sprouts. Cook 10 minutes till crisp yet tender.
- Then mix in cinnamon, thyme, garlic, and apples. Cook 30 seconds, then pour in ½ of broth. Heat to boiling, then add reserved chicken, and rest of broth. Mix in bacon and serve!

Creamy Lemon Chicken with Asparagus and Mushrooms

Ingredients
- Salt
- Zest of 1 lemon
- Juice of 1 lemon
- ¾ C. coconut milk
- 8 ounces sliced mushrooms
- 8 asparagus spears, sliced into 1" chunks
- 3 cloves crushed garlic
- 2 tbsp. coconut oil
- 3-4 chicken breasts

Instructions

- Heat skillet with 1 tbsp coconut oil. Put chicken breasts in pan, heating 3 minutes on each side. Remove chicken and set to the side.
- Toss mushrooms, asparagus, and garlic in same pan. Sauté till asparagus becomes crisp and mushrooms are softened.
- Return chicken to pan and add lemon zest, lemon juice, and coconut milk. Heat to boiling and lower heat to simmer 3-4 minutes till chicken is thoroughly cooked.
- Serve with zoodles!

Baked Chicken Parmesan

Ingredients
- Pepper and salt
- 4 zucchinis
- 1 mozzarella ball
- 1 C. tomato sauce
- 28 ounce can crushed tomatoes
- 2 tbsp. basil
- 2 tbsp. parsley
- 1 diced carrot
- 3 minced cloves garlic
- 1 chopped onion
- 1 C. almond flour
- 2 tbsp. olive oil
- 1 egg
- 4 boneless skinless chicken thighs

Instructions
- Heat olive oil in pan. Add carrot, garlic, and onion to pan. Sauté 3-5 minutes. Pour in basil, parsley, tomato sauce, and crushed tomatoes. Simmer 10 minutes, seasoning with pepper and salt. Take off heat.
- Ensure oven is preheated to 350 degrees. With parchment paper, line a tray.
- On a plate, pour almond flour. In a shallow dish, crack and whisk egg.
- Dip chicken thighs into egg and dredge in flour. Place on tray and season with pepper and salt.
- Cut zucchini into zoodles with spiralizer.
- Bake chicken 17 minutes. Pour ½ cup marinara over each and put mozzarella on top. Bake another 3-5 minutes to melt cheese.
- Serve over warmed zucchini noodles!

CHAPTER 4: DESSERTS

Paleo No-Bake Chocolate Chip Cookies

Your days of feeling guilty about consuming a delightful treat are over. The Paleo diet has come through for you yet again, in ways that many thought would be impossible. Think back to your childhood. Chances are your favorite memories centered on a freshly baked chocolate chip cookie. This is true for many people, and sadly, the Paleo diet does not allow for grains, which many thought meant the end of those memories.

However, just because this is called the caveman diet, does not mean you are stuck with twigs and berries. You can enjoy chocolate chip cookies just as you did as a child.

The best part is, not only are these cookies healthier for you, but they are also easier to make as well! So less time from start to tummy!

The traditional cookies would make even the beginner paleo fanatic gasp in horror. Margarine, flour, and sugar are seemingly the enemy! How could anyone make this recipe into something acceptable?

Fear not! This is a recipe that will blow your mind. It is simple, delicious, and doesn't break the rules. Not even the slightest bit. If you are a rebel but want to stick with the diet, this is definitely the treat for you!

How in the world can something so delicious be so acceptable? Well, replace the flour and butter with Almond butter and flax seed, and you have yourself some acceptable dough components. Throw in some dark chocolate instead of semi-sweet chocolate, and you have yourself a winner!

Ingredients
- 1 c. Almond butter
- 1/2 c. Unsweetened coconut flakes
- 1/4 c. Coconut oil (melted)
- 1/4 c. Ground flax seed
- 1/2 c. Dark chocolate chips
- 1/2 tsp salt (Sea salt)

Instructions
- Take all of your ingredients, and mix them together in a large bowl. Then line a cookie sheet with parchment paper, and roll the dough into balls. Press the balls out on the parchment paper.
- Chill until ready to serve.

Chocolate Brownies

Not only can you have cookies, but you can also have brownies too! This may be mind-boggling, but trust me, no one is pulling your chain. These decadent, chocolatey, delicious brownies are totally paleo friendly and will leave your pallet satisfied, and your sweet tooth happy. Who doesn't like a bit of chocolate every now and then?

Ingredients
- 1/4 c. and 3 tbsp Coconut flour
- 1/2 c. pure Cocoa powder
- 1/2 c. and 2 tbsp Ghee
- 3 organic Eggs
- 3/4 c. Honey (agave)
- 2 tsp Pure Vanilla extract
- 1/4 c. Natural chocolate chunks. (No milk or artificially sweetened chocolate. i.e., Hershey's)

Instructions
- Preheat oven up to 350 degrees Fahrenheit
- Grease up a baking sheet (8x8)
- Using a large bowl, whisk together your coconut flour and cocoa powder.
- Add the next four ingredients and let sit for five minutes. The reason you need to let it sit is it takes coconut flour longer than regular flour to absorb liquid, so you have to give it time to do so to get the proper consistency.
- Add in the chocolate chips.
- Pour the batter, or spoon it, into the pre-greased baking sheet.
- It should take about thirty to forty minutes for the brownies to cook completely. Test their doneness by sticking a toothpick in the center. If it comes out clean, they are done.
- Remove brownies from oven, and let cool completely before you serve them.

Grilled Peaches with Cardamom Creme

Not all desserts have to be chocolate. You can make this dish for a wonderful summertime dessert that would lovely pair with a lamb dish. To make the coconut cream, simply refrigerate a can of coconut milk (full fat) and wait for the cream to separate, then scoop it from the top. Bada bing, ready to throw onto some cooked peaches.

Ingredients
* 2 Ripe, halved and pitted peaches
* 1/2 c. Coconut cream
* 1/4 c. Slivered almonds
* 2 tbsp of Honey
* 1/4 tsp of Ground cardamom

Instructions
* Stir the last two ingredients together in a small bowl. Set these aside
* Fire up the grill over a medium-low heat
* Lay the peach halves cut side down on the grill
* After five minutes, remove the now soft, grill lined peaches
* Place said peaches in a bowl, and dollop some cream on top.
* Drizzle with the mixture you made in the first step, and top with extra ground cardamom, if so desired
* To add an extra element, top with slivered almonds before serving.

Pumpkin Hummus

Cashews make a great alternative to chickpeas. Chickpeas are a no go in the paleo diet which makes hummus something hard to fit in. However, if you love hummus, there is no need to fret. This recipe is completely paleo friendly.

Ingredients
* 1/2 c. raw cashews
* 1/2 c. pumpkin puree

- 2 tbsp of tahini
- 2 tbsp of lemon juice
- 1 tbsp of extra virgin olive oil
- 1/4 tsp of salt
- 1/4 tsp of cumin
- 1/8 tsp of cayenne
- 1/2 tsp of pumpkin pie spice
- 1 clove of garlic

Instructions
- You want your cashews soft, so soak them in a bowl of water for about an hour.
- Once the cashews have been soaked, you need to drain and wash them.
- Place the cashews in a food processor with the pumpkin and blend it until smooth
- Throw in the final ingredients and blend until everything is creamy.
- This hummus can be a little dry. So drizzle some olive oil on top before serving. This also gives it a richer flavor.
- Dip fresh veggies, paleo friendly crackers, or even just a spoon in this hummus, and enjoy!

Baked Sweet Potato Chips

Ingredients
- Salt
- 1/3 C. olive oil
- 1 ½ pounds sweet potatoes

Instructions
- Ensure oven is preheated to 400 degrees Fahrenheit. With parchment paper, line a tray.
- Slice potatoes using a mandolin slicer.
- Place slices in a bowl and pour olive oil over them. Toss to coat. Arrange slices onto tray.

- Sprinkle with salt. Bake 20-25 minutes till very crisp and golden. Let cool 5 minutes before removing and devouring.

Vanilla Shortbread Energy Balls

Ingredients
- 2 tbsp. water
- Pinch of salt
- ½ tsp. vanilla extract
- ¼ C. vanilla protein powder
- 8 pitted dates
- 1 ½ C. almond flour

Coating:
- 2 tbsp. vanilla protein powder
- ¼ C. almond flour

Instructions
- Mix together all components minus coating ingredients within a food processor. Blend on high till smooth.
- Mix coating ingredients together.
- Make 2 tbsp. sized balls from dough and roll in coating.
- Place coated dough balls onto lined sheet and freeze 1-2 hours till hardened. Enjoy!

CONCLUSION

Thank you for making it to the end of The Complete Paleo Diet Cookbook.

I hope that you found this cookbook helpful in discovering simple yet delicious recipes that will never lead you astray while on the Paleo diet.

Now it is time for you to show the world what you are made of, and put these recipes to good use!

Finally, if you enjoyed this book, please take the time to share your thoughts and post a review on Amazon. It'd be greatly appreciated!

Thank you and good luck!

INDEX

Printed in Great Britain
by Amazon